Nnaemeka Alvan'd Onwukwe
Veronica Nathaniel Umoh

Malaria and Its Visual Effects

The Effect of Malaria on Near Point of Convergence

LAP LAMBERT Academic Publishing

Imprint

Any brand names and product names mentioned in this book are subject to trademark, brand or patent protection and are trademarks or registered trademarks of their respective holders. The use of brand names, product names, common names, trade names, product descriptions etc. even without a particular marking in this work is in no way to be construed to mean that such names may be regarded as unrestricted in respect of trademark and brand protection legislation and could thus be used by anyone.

Cover image: www.ingimage.com

Publisher:
LAP LAMBERT Academic Publishing
is a trademark of
International Book Market Service Ltd., member of OmniScriptum Publishing Group
17 Meldrum Street, Beau Bassin 71504, Mauritius
Printed at: see last page
ISBN: 978-620-2-56429-8

THE EFFECT OF MALARIA ON THE NEAR POINT OF CONVERGENCE AMONG ADULTS IN STATE STAFF CLINIC UYO, AKWA IBOM STATE, NIGERIA.

BY

DR ONWUKWE, NNAEMEKA ALVAN'D

&

DR UMOH, VERONICA NATHANIEL

TABLE OF CONTENTS

CHAPTER ONE

CHAPTER TWO

CHAPTER THREE

CHAPTER FOUR

CHAPTER FIVE

LIST OF TABLES

LIST OF FIGURES

ABSTRACT

Malaria has been reported to affect approximately 300 million people worldwide and 103 endemic countries. A recession in the Near point of convergence (NPC) leads to convergence insufficiency which leads to high exophoria at near and asthenopic symptoms. This study was a prospective experimental research study, carried out to determine the effect of malaria on the near point of convergence among adults aged 18 to 30 years in State Staff Clinic Uyo, Akwa ibom State. A total number of hundred (100) symptomatic patients; 50 males and 50 females were used for this study. The mean NPC during malaria attack was 13.01(break), 15.53(recovery) and standard deviation during malaria attack was 2.111 ± 2.855. Two weeks after recovery from malaria attack, the mean NPC was 9.43(break), 12.13(recovery) and standard deviation was 1.233 ± 1. 561.This caused a recession of 39% in NPC. The mean NPC in subjects with 1+ parasitaemia was -3.25(break), -3.59(recovery) and standard deviation was 1.598 ± 1.551. Those with 2+ parasitaemia had a mean NPC of -3.92 (break), -3.20(recovery) and standard deviation was 1.256 ± 3.600. Measuring the correlation between the NPC before and after recovery from malaria attack using the SPSS statistical package at 0.05 level of significance, P=0.00 which is less than the 0.05 level of significance. Results also showed that the degree of malaria had a significant effect on NPC break (p=0.023) but not on recovery (p=0.487). In conclusion, malaria causes a recession in the NPC.

CHAPTER ONE

1.0 INTRODUCTION

This chapter explains the following: Background to the Study, Statement of Problem, Purpose and Objectives of Study, Significance of the Study. Presented also in this chapter are; Limitations of Study, Research Questions and Hypothesis, Definitions of Terms.

Background to the Study

Malaria is caused by a protozoan parasite of the genus plasmodium. The disease is most commonly spread by an infected female Anopheles mosquito. It is one of the most important parasitic diseases that affect humans with the largest effect in the tropical regions (Eldryd, *et al.*, 2004). The infection usually results from the bite of female *anopheles' mosquitoes*. It can also be transmitted by transfusion of the infected blood or by needle sharing between intravenous drug users. *Plasmodium falciparum* is the most common causative agent. Approximately 300 million people worldwide and 103 endemic countries are affected by malaria. In Sub-Saharan Africa alone, it is currently estimated that there are more than 150 million clinical cases annually and that about 2 million people die from the disease every year. Until date, malaria is still a danger to travellers (Chuka-Okosa & Ike, 2006). *Plasmodium falciparum* causes malignant malaria. It causes the most severe symptoms and result in most fatalities. *Plasmodium vivax* causes benign malaria and can stay in the liver for up to three years and lead to a rare relapse. *Plasmodium ovale* causes benign malaria and is relatively less severe while *Plasmodium falciparum* is responsible for about three quarters of reported malaria cases. Most of these other cases of malaria are caused by *plasmodium vivax* with just a few caused by the other two species. It is possible to get infected with more than one type of plasmodium parasite. Symptoms of malaria include fever, shivering, vomiting, arthralgia (joint pain), anaemia (caused by haemolysis), haemoglobinuria, retinal damage and convulsions (Eldryd, *et al.*, 2004).

Antimalarial drugs like chloroquine, hydroxychloroquine and amiodaquine have effect on the ocular structures and their functions, this include deposits in the corneal epithelium, causing oedema and decreased corneal sensitivity, chloroquine keratopathy and chloroquine retinopathy.

History of Malaria

Malaria is a protozoan parasitic disease and it is reported to be the world's most widespread parasitic infectious disease. It is predominantly found in tropical and subtropical climatic regions of the world and it is more endemic in developing countries (Uzodike & Ndukwe, 2010).

According to the World Malaria Report (2011), malaria is prevalent in 106 countries of the tropical and semitropical world, with 35 countries in central

Africa bearing the highest burden of the disease, some of which resulted in deaths. 2.37 billion people were estimated as being at risk of *plasmodium falciparum* malaria worldwide, out of this number, 42% or almost 1 billion people, lived under extremely low risk of having malaria (Kakkilaya, 2012). Malaria often afflicts populations that are both impoverished and malnourished and a large portion of the burden falls upon the most vulnerable group within the population which are mostly children and pregnant women. Existing evidence strongly suggests that micronutrient deficiencies and general under nutrition increase the burden of malaria morbidity and mortality. Large numbers of children under the age of 5 years usually die of malaria due to nutritional deficiencies that include protein, zinc and vitamin A. Efforts at decreasing the disease in Africa since the turn of millennium have been partially effective, with rates of the disease dropping by an estimated forty percent on the continent (Bhatt, *et al.*, 2015).

Nigeria is known for high prevalence of malaria. Uzodike & Ndukwe (2010), reported that approximately 50% of the Nigerian population suffers from at least one episode of malaria every year and that malaria accounts for over 45% of out-patient visits. This imposes great burden on the country in terms of pain and trauma suffered by victims of malaria as well as loss in man-hour and cost of treatment.

In Nigeria, as in other tropical developing countries, the high level of occurrence of blood-demanding health conditions due to the increase in road accidents,

3

pregnancy-related haemorrhage, armed robbery attacks, hepatitis and human immunodeficiency virus (HIV) increases the transmission of malaria due to transfusion of infected blood (Chigozie, Ogbonnaya & Vincent, 2006).

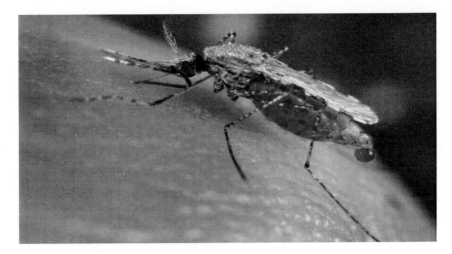

Figure 1.1 – Showing *Anopheles stephensi*

Etiological agents

Malaria is caused by the protozoan parasite of the genus plasmodium. Five of its species cause malaria and they include:

i. *Plasmodium falciparum*

ii. *Plasmodium vivax*

iii. *Plasmodium ovale*

iv. *Plasmodium Malariae*

4

v. *Plasmodium knowlesi*

Plasmodium falciparum accounts for 3 quarter of all malaria causes (Uzodike & Ndukwe, 2010). *Plasmodium falciparum* causes the severe cases of malaria and even deaths. It is generally found in tropical regions, such as Sub-Saharan Africa and South-East Asia, as well as in Western Pacific. Nineteen countries in Africa accounted for 90% of all WHO estimated cases of malaria in 2006 and that more than half of plasmodium falciparum clinical cases occurred in Nigeria, Myanmar (Burma) and India (Kakkilaya, 2012). The parasite invades the red blood cells of all age groups especially young cells. The onset of the infection is insidious, with cough and mild diarrhea, malaise, headache and vomiting and it is often mistaken for influenza. Using the semi quantitative count which depends on the asexual parasites identified in each field. It is recorded as shown below:

1-10 per 100 high power fields.............................1+

11-100 per 100 high power fields.........................2+

1-10 in every high power field.............................3+

More than 10 in every high power field..................4+

The + signifies the percentage of red blood cells that are infected in the blood film (Monica, 2005).

Plasmodium vivax is transmitted in 95 countries in tropical, sub-tropical and temperate regions. It is the only *Plasmodium* parasite that exists in temperate latitudes that stretches up to the Korean peninsula and across the southern temperate latitudes of Asia to the Mediterranean Sea (kakkilaya, 2012). *Plasmodium vivax* causes benign fever (Uzodike & Ndukwe, 2010). It starts with invading the reticulocytes. The fever starts with a rigor, the patient feels cold and temperature rises to about 40 degrees centigrade. After half an hour, the hot or flash phase begins which gives way to profuse perspiration and a gradual fall in temperature. The cycle is repeated after 48 hours. Later, the spleen and liver enlarges and may become tender leading to the development of anaemia slowly.

Plasmodium ovale is found in Africa and sporadically in south east Asia and the western pacific (Kakkilaya, 2012). Its clinical manifestation is the same with *plasmodium vivax* (Stanley, 2006).

Plasmodium malariae is wide spread throughout sub-saharan Africa, Asia, Indonesia, many islands of western pacific and areas of the Amazon basin of South America (Kakkilaya, 2012). Stanley in 2006, reported that it is associated with mild symptoms and bouts of fever every 3rd day. It presents for many years with occasional occurrence of fever or without producing any symptoms. Complications include glomerulo nephritis and nephritic syndrome in children.

Plasmodium knowlesi is primate malaria specie that is being increasingly reported from remote areas of south East Asia from countries such as Malaysia, Thailand, Vietnam, Myanmar and Philippines (Kakkilaya, 2012).

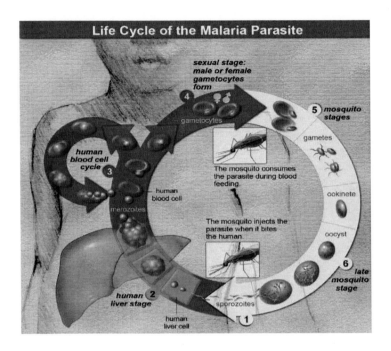

Figure 1.2 – Showing the Life Cycle of the malaria parasite

Table 1.1 – Showing the relationship between the life cycle of malaria parasites and clinical features (Stanley, 2006)

Cycle/Feature	*P. vivax and P. ovale*	*P. malariae*	*P. falciparum*
Minimum incubation	8 – 25 days	15 – 30 days	8 – 25 days

Asexual cycle	48 hours	72 hours	48 hours
Periodicity of fever	Tertian	Quartan	Apenodic
Delayed onset	Common	Rare	Rare
Relapses	Common up to 2 years	Many years later	Up to 1 year

Diagnosis of Malaria

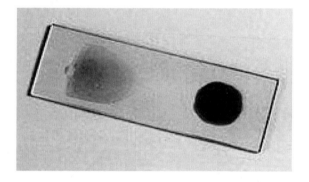

Figure 1.3 – Showing the Blood Sample on a Test Kit

Malaria is better diagnosed using good laboratory facilities and the process involves:

1. Collection of blood sample using a plastic bulb pipette and card with a line on it showing sizes of drops, position of the blood film and area to be covered by the blood film. In preparing the blood film for analysis, a grease

free slide is used and a thick or thin film can be used. The film should have

a smooth tail end and free of vertical lines and holes.

2. Malaria parasites can be identified by examining under the microscope a

drop of the patient's blood, spread out as a "blood smear" on a microscope

slide, prior to examination, the specimen is stained (most often with the

Giemsa stain) to give the parasites a distinctive appearance.

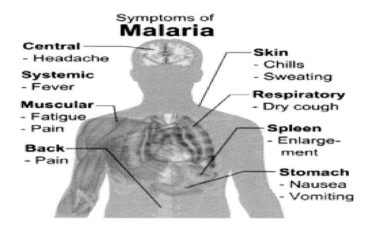

Figure 1.4 – Showing the Clinical Features of Malaria

Malaria is a febrile illness with a wide range of clinical manifestation, from flu

like symptoms that may remain undiagnosed to severe malaria with seizures,

coma and multiple organ failure.

Most of the clinical manifestations are due to individual immunity response (over

production of ill, TNF and other cytokines). Malaria disease can be categorized

as uncomplicated or severe (complicated).

Uncomplicated Malaria

The features include the following;

- Fever

- Chills

- Headache

- Dizziness

- Back pain

- Myalgia, Joint and bone pains

- Cough, Chest pain

- Weakness, Prostration

- Vomiting, Diarrhoea.

Severe (complicated malaria)

The features include the following;

- Prostration

- Hyperpyrexia

- Dehydration

- Hypotension

- Circulatory collapse

- Jaundice

- Coma

- Severe anaemia

- Pulmonary oedema

- Acidosis

- Haemoglobinuria

Control of Malaria

Malaria is a preventable and treatable disease. Interventions to prevent malaria include;

- **Vector control**: This refers to methods used to decrease malaria by reducing the levels of transmission by mosquitoes. For individual protection, the most effective insect repellents are based on DEET or picaridin (Kajfasz, 2009).

- **Insecticide-treated Mosquito Nets (ITNs) and Indoor Residual Spraying (IRS):** This have been shown highly effective in preventing malaria among children in areas where malaria is common (Lengeler, 2004). Tanser, Lengeler & Sharp (2010), Prompt treatment of confirmed cases with artemisinin-based combination therapies (ACTs) may also reduce transmission (Palmer 2012).

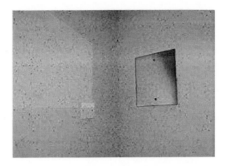

Figure 1.5 – Showing the walls where indoor residual spraying of DDT has been applied. The mosquitoes remain on the wall until they fall down dead on the floor.

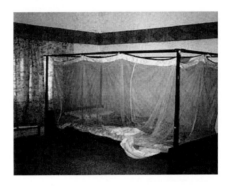

Figure 1.6 –Showing a Mosquito Net in Use.

Mosquito nets help keep mosquitoes away from people and reduce infection rates and transmission of malaria. Nets are not a perfect barrier and are often treated with an insecticide designed to kill the mosquito before it has time to find a way past the net. Insecticide-treated nets are estimated to be twice as effective as untreated nets, and offer greater than 70% protection compared with no net (Raghavendra, *et al.*, 2011). Between 2000 and 2008, the use of ITNs saved the lives of an estimated 250,000 infants in Sub-Saharan Africa (Howitt, *et al.*, 2012). About 13% of households in Sub-Saharan countries owned ITNs in 2007 (Miller, *et al.*, 2007) and 31% of African households were estimated to own at least one ITN in 2008. In 2000, 1.7 million (1.8%) African children living in areas of the world where malaria is common were protected by an ITN. That number increased to 20.3 million (18.5%) African children using ITNs in 2007, leaving 89.6 million children unprotected (Noor, et al., 2009) and to 68% African children using mosquito nets in 2015.According to UNICEF & WHO (2015), most nets are impregnated with pyrethroids, a class of insecticides with low toxicity. They are most effective when used from dusk to dawn. It is recommended to hang a large "bed net" above the centre of a bed and either tuck the edges under the mattress or make sure it is large enough such that it touches the ground (WHO 2002).

Intermittent Preventive Treatment: For pregnant women and infants and seasonal chemoprophylaxis for children 1 – 5 years of age.

Near Point of Convergence

The Near point of convergence (NPC) is the point of intersection of the line of sight when maximum fusional convergence is used. The distance from the middle forehead which is also regarded as the spectacle plane to this point of intersection is the measurement of the near point of convergence (Borish, 2006).

In measurement of the near point of convergence, non-descriptive targets are used such as penlight or another simple target on a tongue depressor to help differentiate fusional (disparity) vergence response from accommodative convergence. The accommodative and vergence subsystem are tightly cross related coupled with an accommodative response accompanied by vergence eye movement. Using an accommodative target, stimulus accommodative demand and convergence will lower the expected values for the near point of convergence and recovery. The near point of convergence is when the patient reports diplopia or when the examiner first observes loss of bifoveal fixation by the outward turning of one eye.

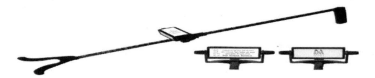

Figure 1.7 –Royal Air Force (RAF) Rule

Binocular Vision Disorders Associated with Convergence

Convergence Excess

A sensorimotor anomaly of the binocular vision system, characterized by a tendency for the eyes to over converge at near.

Signs and Symptoms

14

The signs and symptoms associated with convergence excess are often related to prolonged, visually-demanding, near centred tasks such as reading. They may include, but are not limited to, the following:

1. Asthenopia (eye strain)

2. Headache

3. Avoidance of or inability to sustain near visual task

4. Diplopia

5. Transient blurred vision

6. Abnormal postural adaptation/abnormal working distance

7. Pain in or around the eye

8. Abnormal fatigue

9. Dizziness

Diagnostic Factors

In addition to greater esophoria at near than at distance, convergence excess is characterized by one or more of the following diagnostic findings:

1. High AC/A ratio

2. Low negative or excessive positive fusional vergence ranges

3. Reduced positive relative accommodation (PRA)

4. Eso-fixation disparity with higher than normal associated phoria

5. Inadequate binocular accommodative facility

6. More esophoria at near than far

Treatment

15

Convergence excess is often successfully managed by prescription of therapeutic lenses and/or prisms. However, optometric vision therapy may also be required. Optometric vision therapy usually incorporates the prescription of specific treatments in order to:

1. Normalize associated deficiencies in ocular motor control and accommodation

2. Normalize accommodative/convergence relationship

3. Normalize fusional vergence ranges and facility

4. Reduce or eliminate suppression (reduce or eliminate)

5. Normalize depth judgment and/or stereopsis

6. Integrate binocular function with information processing

Convergence Insufficiency

An anomaly of the binocular vision system, characterized by a tendency for the eyes to under converge at near.

Signs and Symptoms

The signs and symptoms associated with convergence insufficiency are often related to prolonged, visually-demanding, near centered tasks such as reading. They may include, but are not limited to, the following:

1. Diplopia (double vision)

2. Asthenopia (eye strain)

16

3. Transient blurred vision

4. Difficulty sustaining attention to near point tasks

5. Abnormal fatigue

6. Headache

7. Pain in and around the eye

8. Abnormal postural adaptation/abnormal working distance

9. Dizziness

Diagnostic factors

Convergence insufficiency is characterized by one or more of the following diagnostic findings:

1. High exophoria at near

2. More Exophoria at near than far

3. Low Accommodative-Convergence/Accommodation ratio

4. Reduced near-point of convergence   .

5. Low fusional vergence ranges and/or facility

6. Exo-fixation disparity with steep forced vergence slope

1.1 Statement of Problem

It has been observed in recent times that malaria has been a major contributing factor to adults who have difficulty in seeing things that are near. Therefore, this study aims at determining the effect of malaria on the near point of convergence among adults in State Staff Clinic Uyo, Akwa Ibom State.

1.2 Purpose of Study

The purpose of this study is to ascertain the level of change in the near point of convergence during malaria attack among adults.

The objectives of the study include:

- To determine the effect of malaria on the near point of convergence.
- To determine the effect of the severity of malaria parasitaemia on the near point of convergence.
- To establish whether the age of participants influence the effect of malaria on the near point of convergence.
- To establish whether the gender of the participants influence the effect of malaria on the near point of convergence.

1.3 Research Questions and Hypotheses

1.3.1 Research Questions

- What is the effect of malaria on the near point of convergence among adults?

- What is the effect of the severity of malaria parasitaemia on the near point of convergence?

- Does the age of participants influence the effect of malaria on the near point of convergence?

- Does the gender of participant influence the effect of malaria on the near point of convergence?

1.3.2 Research Hypotheses

- There is no significant gender difference on the effect of malaria on the near point of convergence among adults aged 18 – 30 years (P < 0.05).

- There is no significant age difference on the effect of malaria on the near point of convergence among adults aged 18 – 30 years (P < 0.05).

1.4 Significance of the Study

This study will provide data on the effect of malaria on the near point of convergence among adults in State Staff Clinic Uyo, Akwa Ibom state.

This study will add more information to the existing literature on malaria and near point of convergence.

1.5 Limitations of Study

Non adherence to instructions by some adults during the examination procedures may have affected some of the findings. Also the ages of the adults could not be substantiated, they could possibly not have given their actual ages.

1.6 Definition of Terms

Accommodation (eye) – The process by which the eye increases optical power to maintain a clear image (focus) on an object as it draws near.

Anaemia – Is a condition that develops when your blood lacks enough healthy red blood cells or haemoglobin.

Asthenopia – Also known as Eye strain is an eye condition that manifests through nonspecific symptoms such as fatigue, pain in or around the eyes, blurred vision, headache and occasional double vision.

Chloroquine keratopathy – Is an example of drug – induced phospholipidosis. **Chloroquine retinopathy** – This is also known as Bull's eye maculopathy, is a form of toxin retinopathy caused by the antimalarial drugs chloroquine or hydroxychloroquine, which are sometimes used in the treatment of autoimmune disorders such as rheumatoid arthritis and systemic lupus erythematosus.

Coma – Is a deep state of prolonged unconsciousness in which a person cannot be awakened; fails to respond normally to painful stimuli; light, or sound; lacks a normal wake-sleep cycle; and does not initiate voluntary actions.

Convulsion – Is a medical condition where body muscles contract and relax rapidly and repeatedly resulting in an uncontrolled shaking of the body.

Cytokin – Are a broad and loose category of small proteins that are important in cell signalling.

Endemic – A disease or condition regularly found among particular people or in a certain area.

Fever – Also known as hyperthermia, pyrexia, or elevated temperature. It is an abnormally high blood temperature, usually accompanied by shivering, headache and in severe instances, delirium.

Fusion – Also known as synthesis is the process of combining two or more distinct entities into a new whole.

Haemoglobinuria – Is a condition in which the oxygen transport protein haemoglobin is found in abnormally high concentrations in the urine.

Hypoxia – Is a condition in which the body or a region of the body is deprived of adequate oxygen supply at the tissue level.

Insidious –Producing harm in a stealthy, often gradual manner.

Jaundice – A medical condition with yellowing of the skin or whites of the eyes, arising from excess of the pigment bilirubin and typically caused by obstruction of the bile duct, by the liver disease, or by excessive breakdown of red blood cells.

Malignant – A term for diseases in which abnormal cells divide without control and can invade nearby tissues.

Prophylactic – Is a medical or a treatment designed and used to prevent a disease from occurring.

Quartan – A term denoting a mild form of malaria causing a fever that recurs every third day.

Strabismus – Also known as crossed eye; A condition in which the eyes do not properly align with each other when looking at an object.

Tertian – A term denoting a form of malaria causing a fever that recurs every second day.

CHAPTER TWO

2.0 LITERATURE REVIEW

There has been no study on the effect of malaria on the near point of convergence, in State Staff Clinic Uyo, Akwa Ibom State. The following literature reviews are related to previous works on the effect of malaria on the near point of convergence in various populations.

Azuamah, Esenwah & Iwuala (2018), conducted a study on the effects of malaria on near point of convergence of the eye. This study was carried out to determine the effect of malaria on the near point of convergence (NPC) of the eye. One hundred and seventy patients; 54 males and 116 females within the age range of 18-37 years were examined. The mean age of the patients was 22.49±4.4. The mean NPC during malaria attack was 10.62±1.11. Two weeks after recovery from malaria attack, the mean NPC was 7.62±0.69. The result showed a recession of 39.37% in the near point convergence, leading to convergence insufficiency which results in high exophoria at near and asthenopic symptoms of the eye. Measuring the correlation between the NPC during and after recovery from malaria attack with SPSS statistical software using the T-Test at 0.05 level of significance, a significant effect (P<0.05) of malaria on the NPC values was found.

Ahuama, *et al.*, (2015), conducted a research on the effect of Black Tea on Some Visual Functions of young Adults. Black tea which is often taken to alert the mental state of the mind is the fermented category of camellia sinensis plant. It contains theophylline, theaflavin, caffeine, polyphenols, flavonoids, theanine and catechins, and because of the stimulatory effects of these constituent compounds, it affects the central nervous system. This research work was carried out to determine the effects of black tea on some visual functions such as amplitude of accommodation, near point of convergence, pupillary size, lateral phoria at far and near of young adults aged 16-30 years old. 50 subjects were used and baseline measurements of their pupillary size, amplitude of accommodation, near point of convergence and lateral phoria at far and near were taken prior to their consumption of black tea. Measurements were taken again 30, 60 and 90 minutes' post administration of black tea in order to obtain the induced values. From the statistical analysis using t-test, results revealed that black tea slightly increased pupillary size and habitual phoria at near while its effects on amplitude of accommodation, near point of convergence and habitual phoria at far, were not statistically significant. More work should be done using green tea which is not fermented. Also, the middle aged should be used for the study, as this group usually consumes more tea.

Esenwah, Azuamah & Nwabueze (2013), carried out a comparative study on the effect of 1+ and 2+ plasmodium *falciparum* malaria infection on the near point of convergence in Federal University of Technology, Owerri, Imo State, Nigeria and Madonna University Teaching Hospital Elele, Rivers State, Nigeria respectively on One hundred seventy patients diagnosed of having malaria. The age range of the patients was 18 to 37 with a mean age standard deviation of 22.49

± 4.4. After the confirmation of malaria by a medical laboratory scientist, the near point of convergence using push – up method before commencement of treatment was then taken for patients with 1+ and 2+ parasitaemia of the *plasmodium falciparum.* Two weeks after recovery, after which the effect of the malaria drugs had worn off, the second reading of the near point of convergence was taken. Results showed that the mean NPC value for patients with 1+ parasitaemia was 10.44 ± 0.96 cm during malaria attack and reduced to 7.60 ± 0.68 cm after recovery. This resulted in a 37.4% recession in NPC during malaria attack and 7.68 ± 0.72 cm after recovery showing a 41.1% recession in NPC during malaria attack. The SPSS statistical software was used to determine the statistical values of the data such as the mean, standard deviation, standard error mean, range, maximum and minimum values. The null hypothesis was tested using Paired Sample T-TEST at 95% confidence interval and 0.05 level of significance.

Uzodike & Ndukwe (2010), conducted a study on the effect of malaria on the near point of convergence (NPC) and the amplitude of accommodation (AA) using a population of 100 patients from First Rivers Hospital Port Harcourt, Nigeria. The subjects included both sexes of age range 9-38 years. The base data was collected immediately after confirmation of malaria and commencement of treatment. Data collected was stratified into 3 age groups of 10 years' interval (9-18, 19-28, 29-38) with their mean ages and standard deviation. The greater number of subjects was between 19-28 years (46%), 9-18 (22%) and 29-38

(32%). Malaria caused a recession on NPC and the percentage recession decreased with increase in age with age group 9-18 having the greatest recession of 3.05cm (42.07 %) and age group 29-38 having the least recession of 2.75cm (24.345). These effects were statistically significant ($p<0.05$). A decrease was also seen in AA and the percentage reduction increased with increased age. The age group 29-38 had the greatest reduction (-2.09D; 28.79%). The near point of convergence and amplitude of accommodation was taken 2 weeks after taking the anti-malarial drug to allow its effect to be eliminated from the system. The research work showed that malaria causes a recession in near point of convergence and reduction in amplitude of accommodation.

Odjimogho & George (2009), conducted a study on the effect of alcohol on the near point of convergence, amplitude of accommodation and pupil size using 150 non-habitual smokers and drinkers within the age group 20-30 years with a mean age of 24.1±2.8 years. They weighed an average of 70kg and had a light meal to avoid stomach upset during the experiment. Each subject was meant to consume 30ml of brandy (containing 40% alcohol). Measurements were repeated at an interval of 30, 60 and 90 minutes. The result showed that the mean amplitude of accommodation declined slightly while the mean near point of convergence and pupil diameter increased after consumption of alcohol. Statistical analysis using ANOVA showed that the difference between means was statistically significant in amplitude of accommodation, pupil size and the mean near point of convergence.

Ajayi & George (2008), carried out a study on the acute effect of caffeine on Amplitude of accommodation and near point of convergence. Caffeine is widely consumed in kola nuts and in other products in Sub-Saharan Africa. They examined the acute effect of caffeine on the amplitude of accommodation and near point of convergence of healthy Nigerians. Forty volunteers between ages of 20 and 27 years with refractive power$\pm$ 0.50 DS were employed. Amplitude of accommodation (AOA) and Near point of convergence (NPC) were measured at 0, 30, 60 and 90 minutes after the ingestion of coffee by two groups of participants, namely the experimental (caffeinated coffee) and control (decaffeinated coffee) groups. The result showed that ingested caffeine increases mean AOA by almost 2.00D within 30 minutes. The NPC and AOA in the decaffeinated coffee was statically insignificant ($P > 0.05$) within the 0 to 90minutes of ingestion. However, there was a significant increase in the AOA of the experimental group ($P < 0.05$). The result suggests that further studies would be most desirable with the older and larger population.

Igwe, Akunyili & Ikonne (2007), carried out a study on the ocular effects of acute ingestion of Cola nitida (Linn) on healthy adult volunteers? The study was an experimental study where ten healthy adult volunteers of both sexes weighing between 52 and 62 kg (mean 60.2 + 1.5 kg) were used. The ethno

27

pharmacological effects of bolus ingestion of 30g of Cola nitida was investigated on visually acute and healthy volunteers in order to determine its ocular implications or effects. Results showed that Cola nitida had no effect on the pupil diameter, visual acuity and intraocular pressure but improved the near point of convergence by 43% and increased the amplitude of accommodation by 11% while existing heterophorias are ameliorated. The stimulating effect of Cola nitida might overcome asthenopic symptoms with convergence insufficiency and allows near work to be done without stress. Somnolence and ocular muscle imbalance common features of the elderly can be ameliorated or relieved.

Timothy & Chima (2005), conducted a study to know the effect of sulphadoxine and pyrimethamine on habitual lateral phoria and near point of convergence. Hundred volunteers within 18-29 years of age, comprising of both sexes were used in the study. The drug (Fansidar) composed of 500mg sulphadoxine and 25mg of pyrimethamine was administered as a prophylactic to each of the subject. After 4hours (effective period of the drug), the habitual lateral phoria and near point of convergence were again measured at intervals of 15 minutes each for 4 times for each subject and recorded. There was a slight peak increase in exophoria after 30 minutes after which it decreased to its baseline. There was a peak increase of exophoria after 45 minutes' post ingestion of drug with percentage change of 18.2% after which it decreased to mean baseline. Peak increase in near point of convergence was noticed after 45 minutes and the percentage change was 3% of the mean change after which it gradually decreased towards the normal. About 26.6% of the subjects showed an increase in the near point of convergence while 13.3% reported a decrease. About 70% of the subjects showed no change at far for the habitual lateral phoria while 60% showed no change at near.

CHAPTER THREE

3.0 METHODOLOGY

3.1 Ethical Consideration

- The permission to carry out this prospective experimental research study was sought for and obtained first from the Ethical Committee, Department of Optometry, Faculty of Health Sciences, Madonna University Research Project Committee.

- Permission was also obtained from the Assistant Medical Superintendent, State Staff Clinic, Uyo.

- Written consent was obtained from study participants.

- Measures were taken to ensure confidentiality of data.

- The entire study and its procedures were thoroughly explained to the subjects.

3.2 Research Design

This study was a prospective experimental research study carried out in State Staff Clinic Uyo, Akwa Ibom state to determine the effect of malaria on the near point of convergence among adults.

3.3 Study Population

The target populations for this study were the people visiting State Staff Clinic Uyo, Akwa Ibom state. Consisting of; 50 males and 50 female adults, between November 2018 and January 2019.

3.4 Area of Study

This research was carried out in State Staff Clinic Uyo, Akwa Ibom State. It is a clinic in Akwa Ibom State Secretariat (Idongesit Nkanga Secretariat) under the ministry of health, located at IBB Avenue, Uyo, Akwa Ibom State which is under the jurisdiction of Akwa Ibom State. The ministry was formed as MDA (Ministries, Departments and Agencies), in 1987, with the creation of the Nigerian state of Akwa ibom. It has 7 divisions, or directorates, each having their own distinct responsibilities to the ministry and the government.

3.5 Inclusion Criteria and Exclusion Criteria

The inclusion criteria included patients suffering from malaria in State Staff Clinic Uyo, Akwa Ibom State, between the ages of 18 to 30 years who gave their consent.

Patients not suffering from malaria, presbyopic patients, geriatric patients, patients with refractive errors, ocular pathologies and those who did not give their consent for the study were excluded.

3.6 Sample Size and Sampling Technique

The sample size was 100 participants comprising of fifty (50) males and fifty (50) females. The sampling technique used was criterion sampling technique.

3.7 Instrumentation

Instruments used in this study include the following: Snellen chart, Pen torch, Keeler ophthalmoscope and Royal air force rule (RAF Rule).

3.8 Procedure for Data Collection

Criterion sampling method was used to obtain 100 participants comprising of 50 males and 50 females with malaria for this study. The procedure involved in the test was explained to each subject. The age range of the patients was from 18 to 30 years. On confirmation of the presence of malaria parasite (*plasmodium falciparum*) by a medical doctor and laboratory test by a qualified laboratory scientist with the severity of the malaria, detailed case history to rule out the presence of systemic diseases that might affect the near point of convergence was taken from each participants.

An external and internal examination of the eyes with the use of pen torch and Keeler ophthalmoscope respectively was carried out on each participant to rule out the presence of pathologies that can affect the near point of convergence. Measurement of distance visual acuity and pinhole acuity was also carried out on each participant at six meters (6m) using the Snellen's distant chart to rule out refractive errors.

Measurement of the first reading of the near point of convergence using push-up method with the Royal air force (RAF) rule before commencement of treatment was taken for patients with *plasmodium falciparum*. Two weeks after recovery, after which the effect of the malaria drugs must have if not almost worn off; the second reading of the near point of convergence was taken.

3.9 Data Analysis

The data collected from this study was analysed using the Statistical Package for Social Sciences (SPSS) Version 25.0 statistical software package and T-test was used at 95% confidence level.

3.10 Reliability and Validity

The instruments used in this study are recognized and approved by the Optometrists and Dispensing Opticians Registration Board of Nigeria (ODORBN) and World Council of Optometry (WCO).

CHAPTER FOUR

4.0 RESULTS AND DATA ANALYSES

This chapter presents the results of the data analysis carried out to determine the effect of malaria on the near point of convergence in State Staff Clinic Uyo, Akwa Ibom State.

A total of 100 patients participated in this study. They consisted of 50 (50%) males and 50 (50%) females. The participants were aged between 18 and 30 years (mean age for the male and female was 23.67 years). The median for the age was 23.00 years. The severity of malaria 1+ was -3.25 and -3.59 (break and

recovery), while 2+ was -3.92 and -3.20 (break and recovery). The degree of
malaria had a significant effect on NPC break (p=0.023) but not on recovery

	Severity	Frequency	Percentage (%)
Valid	1+	51	51.00
	2+	49	49.00
Total		100	100.00

(p=0.487). The result showed a recession of 39% in NPC.

The results of the data analysis are presented according to the research questions
that guided the study.

Table 4.1 – Showing the Gender Distribution

	Gender	Frequency	Percent (%)
Valid	Male	50	50
	Female	50	50
	Total	100	100

Table 4.3 – Showing the descriptive statistics of Age, NPC, and the effect of Malaria on NPC (difference i.e. after minus before)

Statistics

	Age (years)	NPC (break)	NPC (recovery)	NPC (break)	NPC (recovery)	Difference (break)	Difference (after)
		during malaria	during malaria	after malaria	during malaria		
N Valid	100	100	100	100	100	100	100
Mean	23.67	13.01	15.53	9.43	12.13	-3.58	-3.40
Median	23.00	13.00	16.00	10.00	12.00	-3.00	-3.00
Std. Deviation	3.947	2.111	2.855	1.233	1.561	1.471	2.745
Range	12	7	19	6	5	6	22
Minimum	18	10	1	7	10	-7	-8
Maximum	30	17	20	13	15	-1	14

Testing for the significance of the effect

One-sample T-Test

One-Sample Statistics

	N	Mean	Std. Deviation	Std. Error Mean
Difference (break)	100	-3.58	1.471	.147
Difference (recovery)	100	-3.40	2.745	.275

One-Sample Test

Test Value = 0

	T	df	Sig. (2 tailed)	Mean Difference	95% Confidence Interval of the Difference	
					Lower	Upper
Difference (break)	-24.329	99	.000	-3.580	-3.87	-3.29
Difference (recovery)	-12.386	99	.000	-3.400	-3.94	-2.86

The T-test table above indicated that Malaria had a significant effect on both NPC break (p = 0.000) and recovery (p = 0.000)

Note that a p-value or Sig. ≤ 0.05 indicates a statistically significant effect

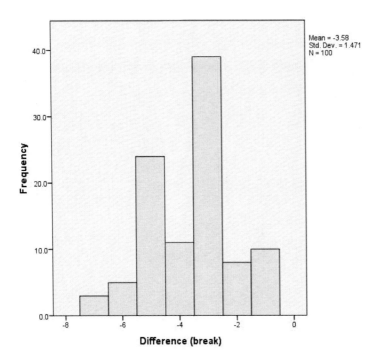

Figure 4.1 – Illustrating the frequency distribution of the effect of malaria on NPC (break)

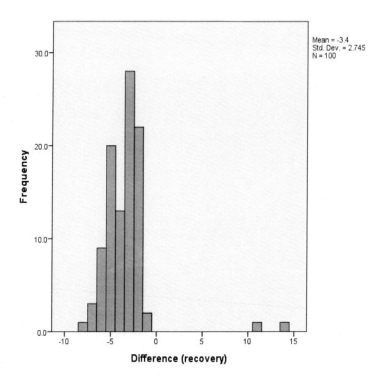

Figure 4.2 – Illustrating the frequency distribution of the effect of malaria on NPC (recovery)

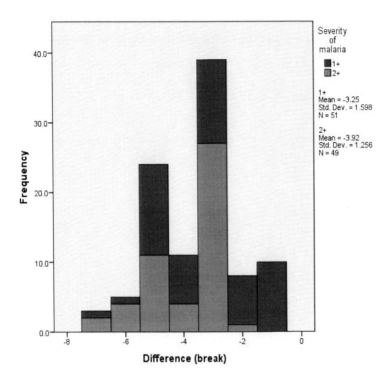

Figure 4.3 – Illustrating if the severity of malaria had an influence on the outcomes (break)

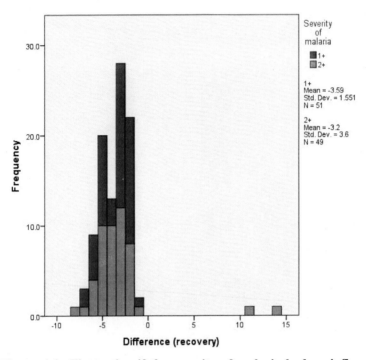

Figure 4.4 –Illustrating if the severity of malaria had an influence on the outcomes (recovery)

Table 4.4 – Showing the group statistics

	Severity of malaria	N	Mean	Std. Deviation	Std. Error Mean
Difference (break)	1+	51	-3.25	1.598	.224
	2+	49	-3.92	1.256	.179
Difference (recovery)	1+	51	-3.59	1.551	.217
	2+	49	-3.20	3.600	.514

For the severity of malaria, 2+ had a higher value of NPC than 1+ but the number of patient with 1+ and 2+ affected the mean making that of 1+ to be higher as seen in figure 4.4 above.

Independent Samples Test

		Levene's Test for Equality of Variances		T – Test for the Equality of Means					95% Confidence Interval of the Difference	
		F	Sig.	T	Df	Sig. (2 tailed)	Mean Diff.	Std. Error Diff.	Lower	Upper
Difference (break)	Equal Variances Assumed	3.123	.080	2.302	98	.023	.663	.288	.092	1.235
	Equal Variances Not Assumed			2.313	94.303		.663	.287	0.094	1.233
Difference (recovery)	Equal Variances Assumed	1.393	.241	-.698	98	.487	-.384	.551	-1.477	.708
	Equal Variances Not Assumed			-.688	64.685	.494	-.384	.558	-1.499	.731

The T-test table above indicated that the severity of Malaria had a significant effect on NPC break (p = 0.023) but not on recovery (p = 0.487)

Influence of gender on the effect of malaria on NPC

Table 4.5 – Showing the group statistics

	Gender	N	Mean	Std. Deviation	Std. Error Mean
Difference (break)	Male	50	-3.46	1.432	.202
	Female	50	-3.70	1.515	.214
Difference (recovery)	Male	50	-3.34	2.904	.411
	Female	50	-3.46	2.605	.368

Independent Samples Test

		Levene's Test for Equality of Variances		T – Test for Equality of Means					95% Confidence Interval of the Difference	
		F	Sig.	T	Df	Sig. (2 tailed)	Mean Diff.	Std. Error Diff.	Lower	Upper
Difference (break)	Equal Variances Assumed	.312	.578	.814	98	.418	.240	.295	-.345	.825
	Equal Variances Not Assumed			.814	97.686	.418	.240	.295	-.345	.825
Difference (recovery)	Equal Variances Assumed	.007	.932	.218	98	.828	.120	.552	-.975	1.215
	Equal Variances Not Assumed			.218	96.863	.828	.120	.552	-.975	1.215

Gender had no influence on the effect of malaria on NPC (p > 0.05)

Hence, it is decided that the null hypothesis that there is no significant gender difference on the effect of malaria on near point of convergence (NPC) among adults (18 to 30 years) is accepted.

Table 4.6 – Showing the relationship between age and the effect of malaria on NPC

Correlations

		Age (years)	Difference (break)	Difference (recovery)
Age (years)	Pearson Correlation	1	-.630**	-.155
	Sig. (2-tailed)		.000	.124
	N	100	100	100

**. Correlation is significant at the 0.01 level (2-tailed).

There was a significant, negative relationship between age and the effect of malaria on NPC (break) only (r = -0.630, p = 0.000). The graphs below show the trends

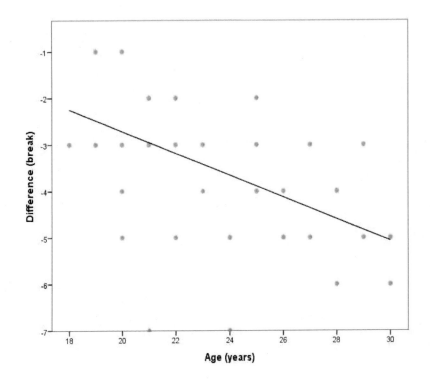

Figure 4.5 – Illustrating the relationship between age and the effect of malaria on NPC (break)

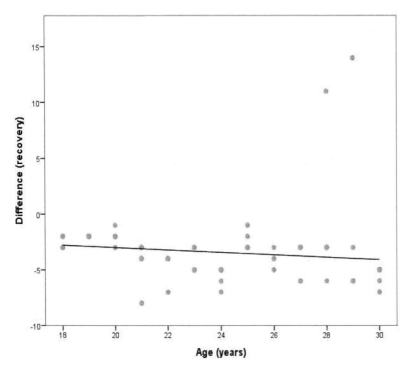

Figure 4.6 – Illustrating the relationship between age and the effect of malaria on NPC (recovery)

CHAPTER FIVE

5.0 DISCUSSION/CONCLUSION/RECOMMENDATIONS

5.1 Discussion

Malaria has been an outstanding problem in developing countries; it has led to many deaths in severe cases. Malaria causes changes in body homeostasis and in respect to the eyes, the changes causes a recession in the near point of convergence value.

Therefore, the aim of this study was to determine the effect of malaria on the near point of convergence among adults in State Staff Clinic, Uyo, Akwa Ibom state. The study population was one hundred (100) people visiting State Staff Clinic Uyo, both males and females. The age of the participants ranged from 18 to 30 years. The study included equal number of participants (50 males and 50 female subjects), age group 18 to 20 years had the highest frequency compared to other age groups.

The result showed a recession of 39% in the near point of convergence with malaria attack, leading to convergence insufficiency which results in high exophoria at near and asthenopic symptoms of the eye. Measuring the correlation between the NPC during and after recovery from malaria attack with SPSS statistical software using the T-Test at 0.05 level of significance, a significant effect ($P<0.05$) of malaria on the NPC values was found (Table 4.3). This finding is in agreement with the work done by Azuamah *et al.*, (2018), who conducted a study on the effects of malaria on near point of convergence using one hundred and seventy patients; 54 males and 116 females within the age range of 18-37 years and found that their result showed a recession of 39.37% in the near point convergence, leading to convergence insufficiency which results in high exophoria at near and asthenopic symptoms of the eye and in measuring the correlation between the NPC during and after recovery from malaria attack with SPSS statistical software using the T-Test at 0.05 level of significance, a significant effect (P<0.05) of malaria on the NPC values was found.

Results also shows that there was a significant, negative relationship between age and the effect of malaria on the near point of convergence (break) only (r = -0.630, p = 0.000) with the age group of 18 to 20 years which had the highest frequency and those within the age group of 28 to 30 years had the least frequency (Table 4.6) which is similar with the study carried out by Uzodike *et al.*, (2010), who found that malaria caused a recession on NPC and the percentage recession decreased with increase in age with age group 9-18 having the greatest recession of 3.05cm (42.07 %) and age group 29-38 having the least recession of 2.75cm (24.345). These effects were statistically significant (p<0.05).

5.2 Conclusion

Results obtained from this study showed that malaria led to a significant decrease in the near point of convergence. Those within the age group of 18 to 20 years had the highest frequency, while those within the age group of 28 to 30 years had the least frequency. From this finding, it can be concluded that malaria causes a recession in the near point of convergence and that its effect on the near point of convergence is not dependent on gender.

5.3 Recommendations of the Study

Based on the observations, analysis and findings from this study, it has shown that malaria causes recession in near point of convergence which might lead to report of asthenopic complaints by the patients during the attack, hence, the following recommendations are given:

- ➢ Eye care practitioners should allow malaria patients to fully recover before carrying out any refractive and binocular vision tests.
- ➢ Public awareness should be created on the effect of malaria on the body.
- ➢ Malaria control measures which include proper diagnosis, promotion of insecticide treated mosquito nets, indoor residual spraying, intermittent preventive treatment for pregnant women and proper treatment should be encouraged especially in the rural areas.

➢ Adequate funding from government and non-governmental organization should be channelled towards the control and treatment of malaria.

➢ However, further studies are recommended on higher parasite load such as 3+ and 4+ parasitaemia.

REFERENCE LIST

Achieving the Malaria MDG target: Reversing the Incidence of Malaria 2000–2015. (2015). *UNICEF. WHO.* Retrieved from https://web.archive.org/web/20160105025916 http://www.unicef.org/publications/files/Achieving the Malaria MDG Target.pdf (accessed June 10, 2019).

Ahuama, O. C., Akubuokwu, E. H., Nwala, O. R. & Ohiri M. O. (2015). The Effect of Black Tea on Some Visual Functions of Young Adults. *International Journal of Research (IJR),* 2, pp. 2348-6848.

Ajayi, O. B. & George, O. G. (2008). Acute Effect of Caffeine on Amplitude of Accommodation and Near Point of Convergence. *West African Journal of Pharmacology and Drugs Research,* 22, pp. 27-30.

Azuamah, Y. C., Esenwah, E. C. & Iwuala, C. C. (2018). Effect of Malaria on the Near Point of Convergence of the Eye. *International Journal of Environmental Health and Human Development,* 14, pp. 9-13.

Bhatt, S. J., Weiss, D., Cameron, E., Bisanzio, D. & Mappin, B. (2015). *The Effect of Malaria Control on Plasmodium Falciparum in Africa Between 2000 and 2015.* Nature, 526(7572), p. 207.

Borish, M. I. (2006). *Borish'ss Clinical Refraction.* Butterworth-Heinemann: Washington, USA, 2nd edition, 4(3), pp. 58-95.

Chigozie, J. U., Ogbonnaya, O. & Vincent, N. (2006). Potential Risk of Induced Malaria by Blood Transfusion in South-eastern Nigeria. *McGill Journal of Medicine,* 9(1), pp. 8-13.

Chuka-Okosa, C. M. & Ike, S. O. (2006). Malaria and the Eye. *Nigerian Journal of Ophthalmology*, 14(2), pp. 3-9.

Eldryd, P., Richard, G., David M. & Geoffrey, G. (2004). Principle of Malaria in Africa. *University of Cambridge Press: Cambridge, England*, 3rd edition, 5(7), pp. 56-98.

Esenwah Emmanuel, C., Azuamah Young, C. & Nwabueze Udochi, I. (2013). Comparative Study of the Effect of 1+ and 2+ Plasmodium Falciparum Malaria Infection on the Near Point of Convergence. *International Journal of Health and Medical Sciences,*1, pp. 1 - 4.

Igwe, S. A., Akunyili, D. N. & Ikonne, E.U. (2007). Ocular Effects of Acute Ingestion of COLA Nitida (Linn) on Healthy Adult Volunteers. *South*, 66(1), pp. 19 – 23.

Kajfasz, P. (2009). Malaria Prevention. *International Maritime Health*, 60(1–2), pp. 67–70.

Kakkilaya, B. S. (2012). World Malaria Burden [pdf] Available online: http://www.malariasite.com/malaria/what is malaria.htm (accessed June 14, 2019).

Lengeler, C. (2004). *Insecticide-treated Bed Nets and Curtains for Preventing Malaria. Cochrane Database of Systematic Reviews*, p. 2.

Miller, JM., Korenromp, EL., Nahlen, BL., W. & Steketee, R. (2007). *Estimating the Number of Insecticide-treated nets Required by African Households to Reach Continent-wide Malaria Coverage targets. Journal of the American Medical Association*, 297(20), pp. 41–50.

Monica, C. (2005). *District Laboratory Practice in Tropical Countries, Cambridge:* University of Cambridge Press: Cambridge, England. 2nd edition, 6, p. 36.

Noor, AM., Mutheu, JJ., Tatem, AJ., Hay, SI., & Snow, RW. (2009). *Insecticide-treated Net Coverage in Africa: Mapping progress in 2000–07.* Lancet, 373(9657), pp. 58–67.

Odjimogho, S. E. & George, C. (2009). The effect of Malaria on the Near Point of Convergence and Amplitude of Accommodation. *The Optometric Educator,* 14(1), pp. 11-15.

Palmer, J. (2012). *WHO gives indoor use of DDT a clean bill of health for controlling Malaria,* pp.10-22.

Raghavendra, K., Barik, TK., Reddy, BP., Sharma, P., & Dash, AP. (2011). *Malaria Vector Control: From past to future. Parasitology,* p. 53.

Stanley, D. (2006). *Davidson's Principle and Practice of Medicine.* Churchill Livingstone: London, England. 2nd edition, 8(2), pp. 40-123.

Timothy, C. O. & Chima, O. U. (2005). Effects of Sulphadioxine and Pyrimethamine on Phoria and Near Point of Convergence. *Journal of Nigerian Optometric Association,* 12, pp. 5-8.

Uzodike, E. B. & Ndukwe, E. K. (2010). Effect of Malaria on the Near Point of Convergence and Amplitude of Accommodation. *Journal of Medicine and Medical Sciences,* 1(11), pp. 539-542.

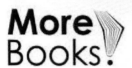
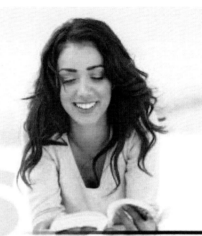
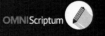

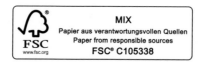